Distribution, publication, and copying in any form are prohibited and subject to damages.

TEN HYPNOSES

Copying, publishing, and sharing with third parties are only permitted with the written consent of the author. Please observe the notes on copyright and usage.

Distribution, publication, and copying in any form are prohibited and subject to damages.

Copying, publishing, and sharing with third parties are only permitted with the written consent of the author. Please observe the notes on copyright and usage.

Distribution, publication, and copying in any form are prohibited and subject to damages.

Ingo Michael Simon

TEN HYPNOSES

48

Restless Legs Syndrome

Copying, publishing, and sharing with third parties are only permitted with the written consent of the author. Please observe the notes on copyright and usage.

Distribution, publication, and copying in any form are prohibited and subject to damages.

© 2024 Ingo Michael Simon
All rights reserved.
Independently published
www.ingosimon.com

Important Notes for Urgent Attention:

The contents of this book are based on the practical experiences of the author with hypnosis applications and psychotherapy in a trance state. Although the author has strived for the utmost care, errors or misunderstandings in the presentation cannot be completely excluded. Therapeutic work with people and the application of hypnosis are solely the responsibility of the hypnotist. It cannot be ruled out that parts of this book may be misunderstood or that the application of a presented procedure may cause an undesirable reaction in the client. The author also assumes no co-responsibility if work with a client is carried out with reference to the statements in this book.

The Author:

Ingo Michael Simon studied psychology and education and is a hypnotherapist with practices in southwestern Germany and Switzerland. With the help of hypnosis-supported psychotherapy, he primarily treats people with persistent psychological conditions. His practice focuses on anxiety disorders, pathological compulsions, and psychosomatic illnesses. His therapeutic offerings mainly include classical and modern hypnosis applications and the dreamland therapy he developed himself.

Copying, publishing, and sharing with third parties are only permitted with the written consent of the author. Please observe the notes on copyright and usage.

Distribution, publication, and copying in any form are prohibited and subject to damages.

INTRODUCTION   **6**

COPYRIGHT AND USAGE   **8**

HYPNOSIS 1   **10**

HYPNOSIS 2   **19**

HYPNOSIS 4   **25**

HYPNOSIS 4   **31**

HYPNOSIS 5   **38**

HYPNOSIS 6   **44**

HYPNOSIS 7   **50**

HYPNOSIS 8   **56**

HYPNOSIS 9   **63**

HYPNOSIS 10   **71**

ALL TITLES IN THE SERIES   **79**

Copying, publishing, and sharing with third parties are only permitted with the written consent of the author. Please observe the notes on copyright and usage.

Introduction

The series "Ten Hypnoses" is very well known in Germany, Austria, and Switzerland as a collection of texts for therapeutic work and is used by numerous psychotherapeutic practices, doctors, therapists, coaches, and other helping professionals. I am pleased to now be able to offer these texts in other countries as well.

Most therapists have their own methods for inducing and deepening trance as well as for exiting trance. Therefore, I have focused on the main part of the hypnosis. The texts in this book can be integrated as the main part into any hypnosis process. The texts in this collection use various hypnosis techniques. I will not explain these in detail, as I assume that users have the appropriate training. It is also not necessary to understand the exact structure or functioning of the different parts. The texts can simply be read aloud, and they will have their effect.

Decide for yourself which text best suits your client or patient at any given time. You can also combine passages from different texts. It is not about using all ten hypnoses in sequence. It is a selection of possibilities.

I want to emphasize that books cannot replace therapy. Psychotherapy or other therapeutic treatments involve much more. A careful diagnosis is the necessary basis for deciding on the use of methods, including whether hypnosis or one of my texts should be used. Even in this case, preparatory discussions, follow-up discussions during the session, and of course, a therapeutic concept for the sequence of sessions and the content approaches are essential parts of therapy. This cannot and should not be achieved with a collection of texts.

In any case, I wish you much success in your work and I am pleased if my text templates can contribute in a small way.

Ingo Michael Simon

Copyright and Usage

Copying, publishing, and sharing with third parties is prohibited and only permitted with the written consent of the author. Please observe the following copyright and usage guidelines.

This work has been carefully crafted and created to the best of the author's knowledge and personal experience. It comprises text templates and application guidelines for professional hypnosis sessions. The author is a licensed psychotherapist with extensive experience in psychotherapy, coaching, and personal training using hypnotic techniques and methods. Nevertheless, the author and the publisher assume no liability for the accuracy of information, instructions, and advice, nor for any typographical errors. The author and publisher accept no responsibility or liability for the application of these texts and recommendations with clients or patients, nor for any potential consequences or unexpected reactions. It is expressly noted that the application of therapeutic and advisory techniques and formulations lies solely and entirely within the responsibility of the practitioner. This also applies to adherence to the boundaries of legally regulated medical and therapeutic practices. The fact that a book containing action proposals is freely available for sale does not imply that its application with clients or patients is permitted for everyone.

Hypnosis 1

... ... You are now going to experience a very deep and healing relaxation ... ... a relaxation that will benefit your body and bring calmness to your thoughts and mood ... ... inner peace and relaxed muscles ... ... inner peace and relaxed legs ... ... inner peace and a relaxed entire body ... ... a calmness that will allow you to relax deeper than a very restful sleep ... ... This is possible because you have already entered a special state of relaxation ... ... You are in trance ... ... and perhaps this trance feels like the moment just before a nap ... ... and in fact, trance is somewhat similar, but in a special way, it is also completely different and far-reaching ... ... because while you can still perceive your surroundings, unlike in sleep, and hear my words, deep within you, special and above all healing changes are happening ... ... For instance, your body may experience a deep healing change, while you are only aware of the outer relaxation of your body, the calmness of your muscles and legs ... ... But your body can relax much deeper ... ... It is already doing so, but the best part is ... ... At the same time, you are experiencing a healing change in your emotions ... ... in your feelings ... ... an inner relief that sets you free ... ... So, your body becomes calm, and your legs become calm ... ... now and whenever you go to sleep ... ...

... ... When you are in trance, images and inner visions become new pathways for your subconscious and for your body, which follows the feeling of these inner images ... ... Perhaps you knew this because you are familiar with hypnosis or because you have learned how and why it works ... ... or you are surprised and intrigued to hear and experience that it actually works exactly like this ... ... You are aware of the difficulties you've had until today ... ... You know the stresses of life that have burdened you and kept your body restless even at night ... ... you have already felt the effects ... ... restless legs ... ... urges to move ... ... tension ... ... But that ends now because you are helping your body to feel the new inner calm and be just as calm at night ... ... You know your goals ... ... You know what you want to achieve ... ... You want to find and experience calm at night again ... ... you want to sleep through the night and dream pleasantly ... ... You want completely relaxed muscles and truly relaxed legs every night ... ... To achieve this, you need to change your thoughts and feelings ... ... When you think about it, you understand very well that a positive and constructive change in your well-being is best achieved when you can let go of disturbing thoughts and feelings ... ... And that is indeed possible ... ... Maybe you are already curious about how this works ... ... It is even possible to activate a balance within you that will help you consistently reach a state of restorative relaxation and deep calmness at night, which regenerates your body and supports every conceivable healing ... ... So, let's begin ... ... Now imagine that each thought is a small, colorful bead in your head ... ... All feelings are also little beads in your head ... ... So, you just need to find and let go of the disturbing thoughts and feelings ... ... and then your body will follow this new relaxation, and your legs will come to rest ... ... your entire body will come to rest ... ... now and every night when you want to sleep ... ... You recognize the thoughts by their color ... ... and your breathing will help you with this ... ... Imagine and feel that with the next breath, the air flows into your head through your nose ... ... It's easy ... ... You feel the air at your nostrils and if you pay close attention, even at the bridge of your nose between your eyes ... ... Then just imagine it flowing upwards ... ... directly into your head ... ... and then harmoniously back to your nose and out ... ... Picture it like this ... ... Your body has already understood this image ... ... Your subconscious has also understood this image ... ... So, let's go ... ... Breathe for your relaxation ... ... Breathe for your relief ... ... Breathe for your recovery ... ... Breathe for your healing ... ...

+++ Variation 1: Restless Legs at Night +++

... ... Let's focus on your legs now ... ... the twitches and movements that you even perform in your sleep ... ... the restlessness and tingling ... ... Perhaps there's even pain in your legs ... ... Maybe you've already tried a lot to calm your legs ... ... Of course, it's best when the body helps itself ... ... Your body is quite capable of helping itself more than it has recently ... ... because there are always conditions within us that can promote the chances of self-healing and regeneration of the body and all its functions ... ... Thoughts and feelings can promote healing ... ... Disturbing thoughts and feelings can also hinder or disrupt self-healing, and such feelings exist within you ... ... It's not your fault ... ... It's the stress and burdens of everyday life that cause this ... ... Imagine that all the thoughts and feelings that have somehow contributed to your restless legs are blue in color ... ... So, in your head, there are many little blue beads that you can let go of to help your body calm your legs ... ... That is possible ... ... In trance, much more is possible than you think ... ... You do this through your breathing ... ... You breathe in and the air flows through your head ... ... You see this in your mind's eye ... ... The air collects all the blue thoughts and feelings and carries them with it ... ... And you breathe them out ... ... As bubbles, they come out of your nose and float through the room ... ... Lots of blue bubbles full of stress and burden ... ... But one bubble after another dissolves ... ... They just pop one after the other ... ... And you keep going ... ... You breathe in and collect all the blue thoughts and feelings ... ... You breathe them out as blue bubbles ... ... They float through the room and dissolve ... ... You repeat this with every breath ... ...

... ... You feel freer and freer ... ... with every breath, freer ... ... And the best part is ... ... Your body has stored this for you and frees you more and more with every breath you take ... ... and deep within, new thoughts are forming ... ...

new thoughts and feelings of inner and outer balance and serenity … … You feel the sensation of inner and outer balance and serenity … … You feel that as you let go of the blue thoughts and with the new balance and serenity, your legs are really becoming calmer and staying calm … … It happens effortlessly … … You just keep breathing and watching the blue bubbles dissolve … …

+++ End of Variation 1 +++

+++ Variation 2: Full-Body Restlessness, Movement Restlessness at Night +++

… … Let's focus on your body now … … the feelings of tension and movement restlessness … … the urge to move at night … … Perhaps there's even pain sometimes … … Maybe you've already tried a lot to calm your body … … Of course, it's best when the body helps itself … … Your body is quite capable of helping itself more than it has recently … … because there are always conditions within us that can promote the chances of self-healing and regeneration of the entire body and all its functions … … Thoughts and feelings can even heal the body … … Disturbing thoughts and feelings can hinder or disrupt these changes, and such feelings exist within you … … It's not your fault … … It's the stress and burdens of everyday life that cause this … … Imagine that all the thoughts and feelings that have somehow contributed to your restless body are blue in color … … So, in your head, there are many little blue beads that you can let go of to help your body relax all your muscles and feel good … … That is possible … … In trance, much more is possible than you think … … You do this through your breathing … … You breathe in and the air flows through your head … … You see this in your mind's eye … … The air collects all the blue thoughts and feelings and carries them with it … … And you breathe them out … … As bubbles, they come out of your nose and float through the room … … Lots of blue bubbles full of tension and restlessness … …

… … But one bubble after another dissolves … … They just pop one after the other … … Tension pops … … Restlessness dissolves … … You breathe in and collect all the blue thoughts and feelings … … You breathe them out as blue bubbles … … They float through the room and dissolve … … You repeat this with every breath … … You feel freer and freer … … with every breath, freer … … And the best part is

… … Your body has stored this for you and frees you more and more with every breath you take … … and deep within, new thoughts are forming … … new thoughts and feelings of inner and outer peace … … thoughts and feelings of deep peace … … You feel that as you let go of the blue thoughts, your entire body is really becoming calmer and staying calm … … It happens effortlessly … … You just keep breathing and watching the blue bubbles dissolve … …

+++ End of Variation 2 +++

… … Now you can let go of the image of the bubbles, as they have already completely dissolved … … and something truly unique has happened … … Disturbing and restless thought patterns have dissolved, but better yet … … New patterns of inner balance have formed … … healing balance within … … healing feelings … … healing confidence … … and with that, the regenerative and self-healing power of your body is fully activated … … and in every moment of conscious rest, your body breathes out all the blue thoughts and feelings if there are any left, and above all … …

… … Every night when you sleep, your body finds all imaginable blue thoughts and feelings and breathes them out … … for your peace … … for your liberation … … for calm legs … … for a calm body … … for true relaxation … … for good sleep … … for you … …

Hypnosis 2

… … You are here today to find peaceful sleep again … … truly peaceful sleep, just like it used to be … … with relaxed muscles, relaxed legs, and a truly relaxed body … … You remember a time of peaceful sleep now … … You know that this time existed, and today it is possible to rediscover the feeling of that time … … Today it is possible to walk the path of peaceful sleep again … … and then to make your sleep from now on like it was before when you could still sleep so well and your body felt good and calm … … so you can lie down again and really fall asleep easily and calmly … … sleep soundly through the night … … You are now preparing for this … … Today, you will succeed in reactivating this peaceful sleep because you are ready for it … … You are truly ready now … …

… … In your mind, you are going on a journey through time and space … … to go back to a time in your life when you could sleep really well, peacefully and motionlessly … … On your journey, you pass through images and memories … … you encounter feelings and thoughts you had before … …

perhaps certain situations in your life come to mind immediately on this journey, and it feels like you are making a quick trip through all the time in your life … … and if you want, you can look at some events or simply move past them and continue your journey, soon arriving in your memory and feeling in a time before the restlessness of the legs and body … … in a time before restless nights … … in a time of sleeping through the night, because this time existed and still exists … … You could sleep more peacefully before, much more peacefully and much deeper … … There may have been times when you could sleep exceptionally well … … other times when you slept less well, but then you managed to return to peaceful sleep … … and on your journey, you are getting closer to that time now … … It is as if you are making a big leap into a time of peaceful sleep, to be able to feel it clearly again today … … You don't need to make any effort for this, you don't need to do anything great or come up with a trick … … you don't even need a clear memory with images … … Just imagine arriving at a time when your legs and body were really relaxed and calm at night, and you could sleep well … … Now … …

… … Now pay attention to your feeling … … to your mood and also to the feeling in your body … … because now the feeling of peaceful sleep is palpable again … … as a memory, because all memories of life remain stored within us … … You could just sleep well at night, you dealt with the worries of the day … … maybe you didn't even have any real worries, and that's why you could sleep so well … … Your body could relax, and your legs were completely calm and motionless at night … … and this memory is still within you … … It is also stored in your body because the body stores every feeling … … Feel where you are … … In what time of your life could you still sleep really peacefully? … … Consider how old you were when you could sleep so well … … Also, think about the environment you are in, where your journey has taken you … … and then go deep into these images or simply into the feeling of that time … … into the feeling of peaceful sleep and calm legs … … of a calm body … … of easy falling asleep and deep sleeping … … into the feeling of gentle sleeping through the night … … into the feeling of a calm night … … a truly peaceful and completely restful night … … You are in your thoughts again in this time … … and this feeling of sleep, this path of good sleep, becomes your path today ... ... because now your body remembers how it was ... ... Now your whole body remembers how it works, to sleep really calmly ... ... You remember deep inside how it works, even and especially in difficult times and with problems to let go at night and fall asleep quickly ... ... and your legs remain calm ... ... and your body remains calm ... ... You simply fall asleep in peace ... ...

... ... Your subconscious brings this inner program of peaceful sleep back to life ... ... because now it is truly possible ... ... Your old peaceful sleep program becomes your new sleep program ... ... your inner self clings to peaceful sleep ... ... and with this peaceful sleep program, you continue your journey ... ... It takes you into the future ... ... You carry the ability of peaceful sleep from the past directly into the future ... ... and your peaceful sleep program is active again ... ... peaceful sleep is available to you again ... ... with peaceful sleep, you go from the present into the future ... ... Now ... ... Now ... ...

+++ Variation 1: Restless Legs at Night +++

… … into a future with peaceful sleep, with calm and relaxed legs … … Now … … Now … … You now look at images of the future … … You imagine and see in your mind's eye how it will be … … Your legs are calm and motionless and feel so gentle and tired … … You see that you can sleep peacefully again, just like before, when it was still normal … … Your legs feel free and loose … … You sleep excellently, with a very calm and gentle feeling in your legs … …

+++ End of Variation 1 +++

+++ Variation 2: Full-Body Restlessness, Movement Restlessness at Night +++

… … into a future of completely relaxed sleep … … with a calm body that feels good … … Now … … You now look at images of the future … … You imagine and see in your mind's eye how it will be … … Your body feels gentle and good and lies completely still while sleeping … … Your legs are calm, and your body is calm … … You see that you can sleep peacefully again … … Your whole body is calm, and you feel the pleasant sensation … … You sleep excellently, with a very calm and gentle feeling throughout your entire body … …

+++ End of Variation 2 +++

… … Let the image of peaceful sleep now become very clear inside, very consciously … … In the near future, you will sleep just as peacefully again … … and with this vision and with much confidence, your journey returns to the present … … with a calm feeling … … with the program of peaceful sleep … … and in your present, already in the coming night, your sleep program will help you … … Your subconscious will already give you the good sleep from before in the coming night … … the good sleep with calm legs and a calm body … …

Hypnosis 4

… … Today, you find a truly deep relaxation for complete recovery and balance of body, mind, and soul … … and for deep rest of your body at night … …

… … Today, you find a truly deep relaxation for complete recovery and balance of body, mind, and soul … … and this relaxation is happening now …

… … Today, you find a truly deep relaxation for complete recovery and balance of body, mind, and soul … … and this trance helps you with that … …

… … Today, you find a truly deep relaxation for complete recovery and balance of body, mind, and soul … … and for this, all words flow into your innermost being …

… … Your thoughts become free and glide like waves … … and you become free and open to a truly deep calmness of your body and for recovery … …

… … Your thoughts become free and glide like waves … … and as you let go of your thoughts, your legs let go, your body lets go … …

… … Your thoughts become free and glide like waves … … and all your muscles and tendons now let go … …

… … Your thoughts become free and glide like waves … … and all tensions in your body dissolve … …

… … You are completely calm, and your self-healing power is activated … … Now … …

+++ Variation 1: Restless Legs at Night +++

… … With each exhale, it becomes calmer within you, and your body becomes tired … … and your body feels as good as in a deep and peaceful sleep … …

… … With each exhale, it becomes calmer within you, and your body becomes tired … … and with that, you also feel that your legs adopt the calmness of your body … …

… … With each exhale, it becomes calmer within you, and your body becomes tired … … and just like in sleep, you let go of all disturbing thoughts and find dreamy calmness … …

...... With each exhale, it becomes calmer within you, and your body becomes tired ...... and just like in sleep, your thoughts become calm and still, pleasantly motionless ......

...... With each exhale, it becomes calmer within you, and your body becomes tired ...... and with each sleep, you let go of everything disturbing and enjoy stillness at night ......

...... You are completely calm, and your self-healing power is activated ...... Now ......

+++ End of Variation 1 +++

+++ Variation 2: Full-Body Restlessness, Movement Restlessness at Night +++

...... With each exhale, it becomes calmer within you, and your body becomes tired ...... and your body relaxes completely, like in a deep and peaceful sleep ......

...... With each exhale, it becomes calmer within you, and your body becomes tired ...... and with that, you also feel that the calmness spreads throughout your entire body ......

… … With each exhale, it becomes calmer within you, and your body becomes tired … … and just like in sleep, you let go of all disturbing thoughts and find dreamy calmness … …

… … With each exhale, it becomes calmer within you, and your body becomes tired … … and just like in sleep, your thoughts become calm and still, your body pleasantly motionless … …

… … With each exhale, it becomes calmer within you, and your body becomes tired … … and with each sleep, you let go of everything disturbing and enjoy the calmness of your body … …

… … You are completely calm, and your self-healing power is activated … … Now … …

+++ End of Variation 2 +++

… … You are filled with a deep sense of inner freedom and healing peace … … and this peace spreads throughout your entire body … …

… … You are filled with a deep sense of inner freedom and healing peace … … and this peace is a balm for your legs and your body … …

… … You are filled with a deep sense of inner freedom and healing peace … … and this state calms your legs and your body … …

… … You are filled with a deep sense of inner freedom and healing peace … … and in this peace, you can let go of everything and be free … …

… … You are completely calm inside, and your self-healing power is activated … … Now …

… … Now you don't have to do anything yourself, no more effort … … because in this healing relaxation, everything happens by itself … … … … Now you don't have to do anything yourself, no more effort … … because if you do nothing now, your self-healing power will be even more activated … … … … Now you don't have to do anything yourself, no more effort … … because with that, you feel the recovery of your body and the freedom of your thoughts … … … … Now you don't have to do anything yourself, no more effort ... ... because you have earned rest, and your body has earned rest and healing ... ...

... ... Now feel the deep calm of trance and feel your body, which is more relaxed than it has been for a long time ... ... and this relaxation you will achieve again and again at night ... ... Now feel the deep calm of trance and feel your body, which is more relaxed than it has been for a long time ... ... and this relaxation gives your body deep rest ... ... Now feel the deep calm of trance and feel your body, which is more relaxed than it has been for a long time ... ... and in this relaxation, your legs and muscles rest ... ... Enjoy the deep calm of trance ... ... Enjoy the calmness of your body ... ...

Hypnosis 4

Instructions for Implementation

A self-hypnosis trigger is a signal that initiates the trance state. With its help, even an inexperienced client can continue working with self-hypnosis at home. Naturally, they can work with simple suggestions that are easy to remember and that we should prepare, or they can use simple visualizations. Triggered self-hypnosis is a very useful tool for giving the client a task to continue therapy at home. This way, the time between sessions in practice is not without therapy; rather, it is continued at home.

Completely self-directed self-hypnosis, without a trigger, is also learnable but requires much time and practice. Setting up the trigger is a fairly simple task and relieves the client from the burden of training in self-directed self-hypnosis. Despite all skepticism, I maintain that it is really not a problem to teach a client simple trigger self-hypnosis. It is no more dangerous than meditation, autogenic training, or yoga. One can safely practice it at home. I have encountered numerous patients in my practice who not only managed self-hypnosis well but also enjoyed it. And if a patient enjoys doing self-hypnosis, however simple the suggestion may seem, it is a very good support for compliance. Discuss the procedure once before the hypnosis and provide the client with a brief, keyword-based list of the self-hypnosis steps, so they have a small guide.

+++ End of Instructions +++

... ... You are familiar with these feelings of restlessness at night ... ... restless legs and perhaps restlessness throughout your whole body, and possibly different types of restlessness from night to night, but always restlessness in your body ... ... A simple and powerful self-hypnosis can help you sleep more peacefully at night and, above all, with a calm and balanced feeling in your body ... ... Today, it's about real self-hypnosis, a hypnosis that you can truly do on your own without any help ... ... It's actually quite simple, and I'll show you how it's done ... ... You're going to learn how it's done ... ... Now you're in trance, so you can easily learn how to do self-hypnosis ...

… … We'll start with the induction of trance … … You can use a codeword for this. It's … … Kuriamba … [Please emphasize this made-up word on the "am" … Kuri-am-ba.] … … Simply make yourself comfortable in bed when you're ready to sleep, just like now … … and then whisper this codeword over and over again until you clearly feel that you're becoming sleepy in your head, and that happens very quickly … … You'll become sleepy very quickly when you whisper … … Kuriamba – Kuriamba – Kuriamba – Kuriamba – Kuriamba – Kuriamba … … and with that, you'll reach a stable and healthy trance state, just like now … … Your codeword … … Kuriamba … … is now deeply embedded in your subconscious … … So you can use it whenever you want to enter trance …

… … Then, you deepen the trance a bit, because in deeper trance, physical relaxation naturally occurs, but there's even more … … In deep trance, you are very close to yourself, and this closeness leads to even deeper relaxation of your body … … You reach this deeper trance by whispering ten times … … I am drifting toward sleep … … Simply whisper … … I am drifting toward sleep once … … I am drifting toward sleep twice … … I am drifting toward sleep three times … …

and so on ... ... until you finally reach ten and whisper ... ... I am drifting toward sleep ten times ... ... and with that, you'll enter this deeper trance where you truly find physical relaxation and ... ... feel deeply connected to yourself ... ... The trance you achieve is really deep and pleasant ... ... just like now ... ... You are in complete safety ... ... and can control everything yourself ... ... It's very easy because you're learning it now ...

[For deepening and the main section, I recommend counting the suggestions ... once ... twice, etc. This has the advantage that the client is not distracted by wondering how many times they've repeated the suggestion. It doesn't really matter whether they repeat it ten times. In trance, they can keep track more easily this way. You can also speak all ten repetitions yourself. After all, you are also acting suggestively in this hypnosis. It is not just self-hypnosis training but also a hypnosis session.]

... ... Then follows the main part of your self-hypnosis ... ... The main part primarily helps you postpone all efforts and unfinished business until the next day and experience peace during the night, real peace ... ... You speak a suggestion that frees you during the night ... ... You simply whisper it ten times in a row ... ...

+++ Variant 1: Restless Legs at Night +++

... ... I let all worries rest and continue tomorrow ... ... Again, you count while doing so ... ... You say ... ... I let all worries rest once and continue tomorrow ... ... I let all worries rest twice and continue tomorrow ... ... I let all worries rest three times and continue tomorrow ... ... until you reach ten and finally say and feel ... ... I let all worries rest ten times and continue tomorrow ... ... and then you feel your legs becoming more and more relaxed and comfortable, and you slowly drift off to sleep ... ...

+++ End of Variant 1 +++

+++ Variant 2: Full Body Restlessness, Movement Restlessness at Night +++

... ... I let my body rest and remain still until morning ... ... Again, you count while doing so ... ... You say ... ... I let my body rest once and remain still until morning ... ... I let my body rest twice and remain still until morning … … I let my body rest three times and remain still until morning … … until you reach ten and finally say and feel … … I let my body rest ten times and remain still until morning … … and then you feel your legs becoming more and more relaxed and comfortable, and you slowly drift off to sleep … …

+++ End of Variant 2 +++

[Here we make an exception and skip the awakening phase. The client should perform the self-hypnosis right before falling asleep and simply transition into sleep. This is safe and straightforward.]

… … and then you simply surrender to the pull of sleep … … You simply let yourself drift into sleep, sinking deeper until you sleep … … It's very easy … … You feel the sleepiness and just let go … … Then you fall asleep and sleep until the next morning … … This sleep is healthy and healing … … This sleep helps you experience a truly peaceful night … … and more and more peaceful nights … … So, just fall asleep …

… … Now you've learned how self-hypnosis works … … You can practice it every evening … … When you're tired and ready to sleep, make yourself comfortable in your bed and do your self-hypnosis … … You've learned how to safely and reliably enter trance with your codeword, and you know how to proceed … … Your codeword … Kuriamba … brings you into trance, which you deepen with the words … … I am drifting toward sleep once, twice, and so on … … Then follows your suggestion … … {Here, insert the chosen suggestion from the main part} … … This suggestion gives you peace for the whole night … … At the end of self-hypnosis, you simply follow the pull of sleep and drift off … …

Hypnosis 5

… … You have the goal of achieving clear and lasting peace and relaxation in your legs and body at night … … a noticeable freedom and loosening of your muscles … … Every person has the potential for self-healing within them … … Self-healing that can often achieve much more than many think … … When these inner forces are properly aligned, much faster and more intense regeneration and recovery are possible … … yes, even the calming and soothing of your legs and body at night … … and that's why these inner forces also help you to repeatedly find inner and outer balance in life … … for peace and relaxation … … for calm legs … …

… … Perhaps you've heard before that a single thought can change physical and psychological processes … … That's true … … When we think of something special that touches us deeply, the tension in our muscles changes … … and worries can bring us restlessness and impulses to move even in sleep … … You know this from the restlessness at night … … But it works the other way around too … … A good thought ... ... a special phrase can change your body and your feelings, can bring relaxation and deep peace, and even lasting calm for a restful and good sleep with calm legs and a resting body ... ... You can use a special thought as an affirmation ... ... An affirmation is like a formula that helps you repeatedly ... ... With such a formula, you can always support your body and your emotions in optimizing all healthy and healing processes, and the best part is ... ... Much more is possible than you think ... ...

... ... Now simply rest in your trance ... ... It has a calming effect on your thoughts and your body, especially your legs, and it helps you to truly relax both your thoughts and your body ... ... and you could really use physical relaxation ... ... calm legs ... ... calm and resting muscles ... ... with a pleasant feeling of tiredness ... ... In peace, your body can optimize all processes of relief and healing ... ... Your body can do that ... ... It can do that anytime if it's allowed to perform this important work in true inner peace ... ... and you can help it today ... ... Now it's easy because you're really relaxed, and your legs are completely calm too ... ... and your body can now handle everything optimally ... ... for restful sleep ... ... for a restful body in restful sleep ... ... for resting legs ... ... for resting muscles ... ... for a completely balanced body feeling ... ...

... ... The affirmation you now hear will become that one thought that repeatedly relaxes your muscles at night ... ... for good sleep ... ... for your good sleep ... ... You hear and say internally ... {5-10 seconds pause} ... ... {Read the affirmations a little slower and louder than the rest of the text, and pause for 5-10 seconds after the affirmation before continuing!} ...

+++ Variant 1: Restless Legs at Night +++

... ... I enjoy the harmony of my emotions and the calm of my legs and look forward to every upcoming peaceful and restful night ... ...

+++ End of Variant 1 +++

+++ Variant 2: Full Body Restlessness, Movement Restlessness at Night +++

… … I enjoy the harmony of my emotions and the calm of my entire body and look forward to every upcoming peaceful and gentle night … …

+++ End of Variant 2 +++

… … And now simply enjoy the peace, because that's how the heard affirmation becomes your inner attitude … … that's how the heard affirmation becomes the attitude of your body, especially your legs and muscles, and also … … the attitude of your inner core … … because you've made this phrase your own … … because you've heard it in trance and made it your special belief … … a belief that expresses your intention, your goal, and your will … … but even more than that … … It expresses your willingness … … This affirmation expresses what you are truly willing to do … … deep down willing … … willing for deep peace … …

… … Your affirmation now acts as the deep attitude of your body and your thoughts … … as the deep attitude of your entire being … … The affirmation of physical calm … … the affirmation of calm legs … … the affirmation of inner calm sounds like your inner voice …

+++ Variant 1: Restless Legs at Night +++

… … I enjoy the harmony of my emotions and the calm of my legs and look forward to every upcoming peaceful and restful night … …

+++ End of Variant 1 +++

+++ Variant 2: Full Body Restlessness, Movement Restlessness at Night +++

… … I enjoy the harmony of my emotions and the calm of my entire body and look forward to every upcoming peaceful and gentle night … …

+++ End of Variant 2 +++

… … Allow this inner voice to now unfold its best possible effect … … Significant relaxation and calming of your body has already been achieved … … You now feel the peace within and the peace of your body … … You now feel the calm of your muscles and the calm of your legs … … That's how it should be and that's how it will be every night … … every night calm muscles … … every night calm legs … …

Whenever you hear the affirmation or say it yourself, you are assured … … You experience a peaceful night with good sleep … … You experience a peaceful night with good sleep … …

Hypnosis 6

... ... You focus inwardly on the feeling of relaxation in trance ... ... because this way, your body can truly relax, and you come into a peaceful state of mind ... ...

... ... At the same time, you are open to the words that accompany you on this journey ... ... because this way, your body can truly relax, and you come into a peaceful state of mind ... ...

... ... You turn your mindful attention to your body feeling ... ... because this way, your body can truly relax, and you come into a peaceful state of mind ... ...

... ... And just as mindfully, you follow the words that accompany you ... ... because this way, your body can truly relax, and you come into a peaceful state of mind ... ...

... ... You now think only of health and freedom ... ... and with this thought, you also feel the ever-deepening, healing peace of your legs and muscles ... ...

...... You now think only of deep sleep ...... and with this thought, you also feel the ever-deepening, healing peace of your legs and muscles ......

...... You concentrate entirely on peaceful sleep ...... and with this thought, you also feel the ever-deepening, healing peace of your legs and muscles ......

...... This turns the thought into a feeling of peace ...... and with this thought, you also feel the ever-deepening, healing peace of your legs and muscles ......

...... Deep, healing peace fills your body and your thoughts ...... Now ......

+++ Variant 1: Restless Legs at Night +++

...... You feel your body and consciously perceive it now ...... and this mindfulness allows your body and your legs to rest very deeply and securely now and at night ......

...... You give yourself peace and recovery with this hypnosis ...... and this mindfulness allows your body and your legs to rest very deeply and securely now and at night ......

… … You breathe calmly and evenly for inner balance and freedom … … and this mindfulness allows your body and your legs to rest very deeply and securely now and at night … …

… … You consciously experience inner relief and liberation now … … and this mindfulness allows your body and your legs to rest very deeply and securely now and at night … …

… … Deep, healing peace fills your body and your thoughts … … Now … …

+++ End of Variant 1 +++

+++ Variant 2: Full Body Restlessness, Movement Restlessness at Night +++

… … You feel your body and consciously perceive it now … … and this focus allows your body to become more and more still and gently rest … …

… … You give yourself peace and recovery with this hypnosis … … and this focus allows your body to become more and more still and gently rest … …

… … You have accepted all the helpful words today … … and that's why your body and thoughts have found healing peace and true recovery … …

… … You have truly understood the helpful words … … and that's why your body and thoughts have found healing peace and true recovery … …

… … The helpful words are already deeply anchored in you … … and that's why your body and thoughts have found healing peace and true recovery … …

… … You have walked a mindful path of peace and will continue to do so every evening … … for good sleep … … for good sleep with calm muscles … … for calm and relaxed legs at night … …

Hypnosis 7

… … You know what it's like when you wake up at night or can't fall asleep because your legs feel restless … … And now you want to change that, to become inwardly calmer … … as calm as possible … … with a good feeling in your body … …

… … Today, deep within yourself, you find a helping force … … A force that will help you calm your legs as much as possible … … To do this, you focus your mindfulness today on the helping side of your body, because that side also exists … … So today, you speak to your body … … You enter into this direct contact and focus your mindfulness on all the things your body has already done for you … … You thank your body today for everything that has worked well until now … … Also, for being able to help and for helping you calm your legs … …

… … First, you direct your attention to your hands … … You thank them for always having grasped … … They have often held on, often let go … … They perform their daily tasks as best they can … … They can also give you signals when you should let go inwardly ... ... Pay attention to the feeling in your hands ... ... They signal when you can let go, even of what may have made you restless ... ...

... ... Then you speak to your arms ... ... They hold your hands and lift burdens ... ... You know how heavy burdens are to carry, inwardly and outwardly ... ... Your arms have always helped with that ... ... You thank them now, and they will continue to help you ... ...

... ... Next, you turn to your back ... ... It carries many burdens ... ... It also keeps your body upright and straight ... ... Your back has often served you well ... ... It has functioned well all these years without complaint ... ... You thank it for its loyal service ... ...

... ... Then you speak to your internal organs ... ... You thank them for always doing their work so well ... ... The interplay of all organs enables life ... ... And each organ has always tried to contribute its best ... ... They work like a chain and pull together ... ... But sometimes, a chain breaks or can no longer work as strongly because one link has become weaker ... ...

... ... Then you address your heart ... ... It constantly pumps blood through your body, supplying all organs with oxygen and life ... ... You thank your heart for beating all these years ... ... without pause ... ... in quiet and also in stormy moments ... ... It always works and only rests in the small pauses between beats ... ... Your source of life ... ...

... ... Then you turn to your skin ... ... This large organ is so often overlooked ... ... Sometimes, we take it for granted that it's there ... ... But today, it's different ... ... Today, you thank your skin ... ... for protecting and warming you ... ... for shielding your bones and insides from attacks ... ... for taking on dirt and washing it away, keeping your inner self clean and clear ... ...

+++ Variant 1: Restless Legs at Night +++

... ... Finally, you focus your mindfulness on your legs ... ... You thank them ... ... for carrying your body all this time ... ... They carry the body, keep it upright, and move you from one place to another ... ... They have helped you to be faster sometimes ... ... They accompany you faithfully and helpfully ... ... You also thank your legs for trying to tell you something with their nighttime restlessness … … They have shown you your inner restlessness … … Even if you hadn't understood why it was there, it was still an important signal for you … … Now, you process these signals in your feelings, and your legs are allowed to rest … … and to be calm and remain calm every night … … You allow your legs to rest at night and while sleeping because you can now carefully take care of your inner peace … … because you've understood that it was always about inner restlessness and, therefore, also about inner peace, which you want to achieve and can achieve … … inner peace for calm legs at night … …

+++ End of Variant 1 +++

+++ Variant 2: Full Body Restlessness, Movement Restlessness at Night +++

… … Finally, you focus your mindfulness on the interplay of all body parts … … on your musculoskeletal system, your muscles, and the feeling on and under the skin … … and deep within … … You thank your body for the nighttime restlessness, for the urge to move and get up … … Your body mirrored your deep inner restlessness to you … … Even if you hadn't understood why it was there, it was still an important signal for you … … Now, you process these signals in your feelings, and your body is allowed to find peace at night … … and to be calm and remain calm every night … … You allow your body to rest at night and while sleeping because you can now carefully take care of your inner peace … … because you've understood that it was always about inner restlessness and, therefore, also about inner peace, which you want to achieve and can achieve … … inner peace for a calm and gentle body feeling at night … …

+++ End of Variant 2 +++

… … Then, you grant yourself some more rest … … You let your body rest and trust in its help … … Likewise, you promise your body your help … … You make a pact with your body … … You assure your body that you will do everything to understand your own deep feelings … … To recognize your thought patterns and actions … … to change all of that, to resolve all entanglements, and to be free … … free for real peace at night … … You want to take more mindful care of your own emotional needs … … In return, your whole body strives to become calmer at night, as quickly as possible, because that's truly possible … … This shall be your pact … … And the more you are ready for inner clarity, the more you let go of old entanglements and patterns … … the more your legs strive to truly be calm and remain calm … …

Hypnosis 8

... ... In today's trance, you find help and support from your deep unconscious for achieving your goals as quickly as possible ... ... for achieving deep and lasting relaxation and relief in your legs and body ... ... for reducing restlessness and pressure or even pain ... ... this is your physical and mental healing ... ... Your conscious mind only needs to allow your deep unconscious, with its kindness and goodwill, to help you ... ... and your conscious mind is sure to grant that permission willingly ... ... You certainly grant it willingly ... ... It's very easy; you just need to think ... ... Yes, I want my deep unconscious with all its best strength and goodwill to help me now ... ... Yes, I want my deep unconscious to hear and accept the following words and suggestions exactly ... ... Yes, I want my deep unconscious to process all words and suggestions optimally for my benefit ... ... That's all it takes ... ... If you can agree with these thoughts because they truly align with your will and your goals ... ... then you also agree with the following thoughts and words, which then become your thoughts and words ... ... become your own words ... ... Then you think and say to yourself ... ...

... ... I recognize that my own thoughts can limit or expand my possibilities ... ... and therefore, I focus on expanding my possibilities, on my great chance to finally experience restful sleep ... ...

... ... So I consciously and deliberately direct my thoughts and expectations towards my goals ... ... towards achieving and optimizing a peaceful body feeling, especially in the legs and muscles ... ... for good sleep ... ...

... ... I am already looking forward to the coming days of improvement and relief from my symptoms ... ... and I am happy that I will soon feel better both physically and mentally, and experience relief and recovery ... ...

... ... Truly remarkable how this trance, with its good thoughts and words, now and every night, allows my legs and my entire body to come to rest ... ...

... ... I know very well that body and emotions are connected ... ... and that's why I also take care of both with mindfulness and devotion, and I am mindful of my body and my feelings ... ...

… … So I consciously take care of my body and pay attention to a proper balance between physical exertion and real rest … … and thus, I allow and help my body to bring all internal functions into a natural and healthy rhythm, especially for a truly calm body … …

… … I breathe deeply and consciously in and slowly and long out … … and I feel how all disturbing and worrying thoughts fall away from me, and how I internally adjust to consciously breathing every day for my inner balance and for a calm body at night … … Yes, for a sense of well-being in my legs … …

+++ Variant 1: Restless Legs at Night +++

… … I turn my gaze inward and find within me many feelings that want to come out, and I allow every feeling I discover … … and I feel that allowing and releasing my deep-seated feelings is like an inner liberation and relief, and that this calms my legs, because I don't have to do anything in my sleep, I don't have to run … …

… … I let go of every responsibility that does not belong to me from now on or give it back … … and I feel that I am much freer and healthier when I carry less responsibility, especially when I no longer take on others' responsibilities … … I carry only the responsibility for my health because I truly deserve that … …

… … I accept that not everything can be as fast and as perfect as I would like it to be … … and I resolve to treat myself generously from now on when I can't or don't want to meet the demands of perfection, and I know that this positive and constructive attitude helps me on my path to new and natural health … …

… … I am sure and already look forward to my nervousness and also my inner restlessness in my legs soon dissolving … … because I know that my body recovers, and with it, my inner feelings, my moods, and emotions … … I only walk during the day … … At night, my legs rest … …

+++ End of Variant 1 +++

+++ Variant 2: Full Body Restlessness, Movement Restlessness at Night +++

... ... I turn my gaze inward and find within me many feelings that want to come out, and I allow every feeling I discover ... ... and I feel that allowing and releasing my deep-seated feelings is like an inner liberation and relief, and that this liberates and calms my body because I don't have to do anything in my sleep, I don't have to hold on, and I don't have to fight or run ... ...

... ... I let go of every responsibility that does not belong to me from now on or give it back ... ... and I feel that I am much freer when I carry less responsibility because many burdens fall away from me and my body ... ... I carry only the responsibility for my health because I truly deserve that ... ...

... ... I accept that not everything can be as fast and as perfect as I would like it to be ... ... and I resolve to treat myself generously from now on when I can't or don't want to meet the demands of perfection, and I know that this positive and constructive attitude helps me on my path to new and natural health ... ...

... ... I am sure and already look forward to my nervousness and also my inner restlessness coming to an end, and that my body feels this relief and calm ... ... because I know that my body recovers, and with it, my inner feelings, my moods, and emotions ... ... I let go, I let go at night ... ... My body becomes calm and still and feels very good ... ...

+++ End of Variant 2 +++

... ... Truly remarkable how this trance, with its good thoughts and words, now and every night, allows my legs and my entire body to come to rest ... ...

... ... I will and I will always take time for myself and my health ... ... and I will consciously let peace settle in the evening ... ...

... ... I pay attention to healthy nutrition and constructive movement during the day ... ... because with this, I support all processes of balance in my body, which then finds even more peace and calm in the evening ... ...

... ... Truly remarkable how this trance, with its good thoughts and words, now and every night, allows my legs and my entire body to come to rest ... ...

... ... Good ... ... You have achieved a lot, you have come very close to your goal ... ... The path you have taken today is truly a very good path ... ... And you continue on this path ... ... The path of this hypnosis is your personal path to peaceful sleep ... ... peaceful legs and a peaceful body ... ... real peace deep inside ... ... for true restful sleep ... ... for deep peace at night ... ... deep peace at night ... ...

Hypnosis 9

... ... Deep inside you lies a place of imagination ... ... But imagination is not what we think up or create ... ... Imagination is not the invention of our mind ... ... True imagination is a deep expression of our feelings ... ... because it is always our feelings that guide what images and stories we imagine ... ... Strictly speaking, we don't imagine them ... ... Strictly speaking, these images and stories come to us ... ... They are suddenly there when we open ourselves to our emotions and our inner truth ... ... They reveal themselves unfiltered and real when we allow them and are ready to accept them ... ... On the way to your inner truth, you now embark on a special journey ... ... into and through your imagination ... ... on a journey into and through your own feelings ... ... I accompany you and show you your feelings ... ... in the inner place where your truth reveals itself and is open to you ... ... in the land of dreams ... ... You are already there ... ... You are in the land of your dreams ... ...

... ... You suddenly find yourself on a path that leads you deeper into the land of dreams ... ... You follow this path that leads you to an old house ... ... It is a large house that looks like an abandoned villa ... ... but nothing can be abandoned or forgotten in the land of dreams; everything here endures time ... ... The door is open, and you enter the old house ... ... And inside, you find three doors that lead to three large rooms ... ... rooms where very specific thoughts and very specific memories are kept ... ... You may even find thoughts that you didn't know before ... ... You can also better understand what is going on inside you and thus find new thoughts ... ... new thoughts that help you sleep more peacefully because your legs and body become calmer at night ... ... Today, you find very important thoughts that help you become calmer inside ... ... and then your legs and your body become calmer ...

... ... You are already doing that today ... ... Today is the first day of calmer nights ... ... You go to the first door, and on this door, there is a sign that says ... ... Room of the Past ... ... You open this room and enter ... ... Images of the past blow past you like the wind ... ... They show themselves briefly, then disappear again ... ... Some images are clearer, some barely recognizable … … But above all, you see images that show you what has most contributed to the development of this restlessness in the past, causing your legs and body to show this restlessness so strongly at night … … The images of the past become clearer and clearer; the wind of time carries them into your room and shows them to you … … Perhaps you expected exactly these images … … Maybe you are also surprised by the images the wind shows you … … You pause, stop, and look at these images, whatever they may show you … … You let them have an effect and feel that feelings are connected to them … …

… … You focus on your legs / on your body and feel that they respond to the images … … You feel the tension in your legs / body, even if your legs / body may feel good right now, you feel that they often react to these images at night … … You know that perhaps there were unfinished matters that the images show you, that you cling more to this time than is good for you … … You make it clear to yourself that you can remember and mourn the past, but you can no longer change it … … So, you resolve to hand over the past to the past and learn constructively from it … … Today, you learn that your legs / your body can remain calm because all of this no longer belongs to your present, because all of this is long over ... ... Then you leave this room and close the door ... ... It's over ... ... It's over ... ...

... ... Then you go to the second door with the sign ... ... Room of the Present ... ... You open it and enter the room ... ... The wind blows images of your current life situation into the room ... ... They show themselves before your eyes, some briefly and others long and clearly ... ... Above all, you see what most contributes to your inner restlessness in your current life situation, causing your legs / your body to show this restlessness at night ... ...

... ... Maybe these are images of events or places ... ... Perhaps the wind also blows images of people into the room that suddenly appear ... ... Everything you see is connected to your restless legs / your restless body ... ... because what you see is unsettling for you ... ... You let the images have an effect and think about the fact that you can steer the present yourself ... ... You determine what is allowed and what is important ... ... Some of what you see may not be that important ... ... Here and today, in your thoughts, in the room of the present, you recognize what is really important ... ...

… … You can identify what is unimportant and decide to let it go … … now let it go … … You focus on the feeling in your legs … … The more you can imagine that you can determine what is important to you, the more you feel the calming of your legs … … You leave this room and close the door … …

… … Then you go to the next door with the sign … … Room of the Future … … You open it and enter … … Here a strong wind blows … … the wind of renewal … … In this room, pleasant light shines, and there is infinite space for you … … Here you can develop new paths and plans … … You have understood what is really important and what you no longer need … … This room belongs only to you … … only to you … … Fill it with your ideas and plans … … with your wishes and visions … … Live only in your room, and your whole body will be calm … … Live only in your room, and your whole body will find deep peace at night … …

… … Then close your eyes and dream a beautiful dream … … You dream a truth-dream of peaceful and still nights … … You dream of being able to sleep through and having a wonderful and gentle feeling in your body … … gentle and calm

+++ Variant 1: Restless Legs at Night +++

… … You have understood deep inside that your legs were so restless because a part of you was clinging to past events … … past events that you may not have fully overcome or that had worn you down … …

… … Deep inside, deep in your feelings, you now have a new access to these events … … new and different … … You don't have to think about it; it happens entirely in the feeling … … because a part of you is and remains in the land of dreams and carefully processes all experiences there for you … … And with that, your deep inner self knows that you don't have to hurry, you don't have to chase after the past … … Your legs may rest at night … … Everything is within you and is processed there … … no more running at night … … only peace … … and trust … …

+++ End of Variant 1 +++

+++ Variant 2: Full Body Restlessness, Movement Restlessness at Night +++

...... You have understood deep inside that your body was so restless at night because a part of you was trying to fight against the past and resist it ...... perhaps against attacks or insults from back then, but that time is over ...... The events from back then had worn you down ...... But as tragic as it may be, you can't change them anymore ...... Deep inside, deep in your feelings, you now have a new access to this past ...... new and different ......

...... You don't have to think about it; it happens entirely in the feeling ...... because a part of you is and remains in the land of dreams and carefully processes all experiences there for you and lets go for you ...... And with that, your deep inner self knows that you no longer have to fight, you no longer have to fend off the past, because it can no longer harm you ...... Your body may rest at night ...... Everything is now gently processed ...... no more fighting at night ...... only peace ...... and trust ......

+++ End of Variant 2 +++

...... Then you think about the fact that the land of dreams is more than just imagination ...... it is your path to yourself … … your path to peaceful sleep with a calm body … … A part of you is always in the land of dreams and helps you because … … the land of dreams lies deep within you … … It has always been there … … I'm just telling you about it … …

Hypnosis 10

Instructions for Implementation

Ideomotorics refers to the phenomenon that our body follows our feelings and thoughts with movements. In everyday life, this following is shown as posture, muscle tension, and movement patterns of a person, which naturally change with mood and thoughts. In trance, ideomotoric signals can be used to gain information that the client cannot actively communicate. The subconscious can, for example, answer questions with an agreed-upon finger signal. Naturally, ideomotoric reactions can also be used suggestively, for example, in arm levitations and catalepsies. An ideomotoric approach strengthens trust in hypnosis and one's ability to change, thus promoting therapy.

+++ End of Instructions +++

… … You want to end the nighttime restlessness today …
… That is possible because a special part of you can do that
… … You can reach this special part of yourself very well in

trance and assign it this task … … In trance, much is possible because in trance, you can directly address your subconscious and assign it the task of letting go of the restlessness … … and thus having calm legs and a calm body … … and sleeping well … … Perhaps you already realize that the nighttime restlessness of your body is a signal from your subconscious … … But it's not about your body … … It's about an invitation from your subconscious to come closer and connect with it … … Then restlessness can leave … … This special part of you, the unconscious or subconscious, then no longer needs restlessness … … so I must speak directly with your subconscious … … You dream in a beautiful fantasy … … Imagine the most beautiful fantasy you can think of … … and stay in this beautiful imagination … … You can understand every word you hear from me, but just stay in your beautiful fantasy and imagine that all thoughts, ideas, and fantasies go to the left … … into your left side … … and you, the subconscious of … [Client's first name] … come to the right and go into the right hand … … and give me a signal with a finger of the right hand as soon as you have managed to reach the hand … … While the conscious mind remains in a beautiful fantasy on the left, you, the subconscious of ... [Client's first name] ... come to the right and move a finger of the right hand ... ...

... [Please be patient and stay with it. Don't worry – finger signals almost always happen! Repeat the request a few times kindly and with some emphasis, and radiate confidence. If you are sure a finger signal will come, it will happen faster than if you doubt.] ...

... ... There is the signal, good ... ... Thank you ... ... Now, subconscious of ... [Client's first name] ... make sure the conscious mind is deeply dreaming on the left side, so we can work well together ... ... The greeting finger should be the yes finger ... ... For every confirmation, you can move it ... ... For rejection, you can move a different finger ... ... Now choose a finger for no and move it ... ... [Wait for finger signal!] ... ... Thank you ... ... We now have the ... [Name the yes finger] ... for yes and the ... [Name the no finger] ... for no ... ... So, we can begin ... ... We can now start to end the nighttime restlessness forever ... ... Are you ready? ... ... [Wait for yes finger!] ... ... Good ... ... so let's begin ... ...

... ... Subconscious of ... [Client's first name] ... we have understood that the physical restlessness at night has causes, but we do not know exactly what they are ... ... I know you are trying to establish better communication with the conscious mind, with the intellect. I also know that the restlessness will disappear if your signals and messages are received differently. I want to help you find a new path without restlessness, and the conscious mind will make an effort in everyday life to be in contact with you with mindfulness ... ... But you have to do it because you, the subconscious of ... [Client's first name] ... can do it ... ... For yes, please use the yes finger, and for no, the agreed-upon no finger ... ... We'll start now ... ...

... ... Now find in the infinite variety of possibilities within you a way of communication with the conscious mind. This path must have nothing to do with physical restlessness. It must allow your entire body to really rest, to rest with a good feeling ... ... Show me with the yes finger as soon as you have found a good path ... ... [Wait for yes finger!] ... ... Good, you have found a new path ... ... But we want to make sure that it works well too ... ... Imagine what it will be like when the conscious mind better understands your signals and needs and handles them carefully ... ... Imagine what it will be like when you manage in your waking everyday life to repeatedly feel and perceive your feelings and take careful care of yourself ... ... Feelings and thoughts together ... ... Emotions and considerations together ...

+++ Variant 1: Restless Legs at Night +++

... ... Subconscious and conscious mind together ... ... and imagine that you ... ... subconscious of... [Client's first name] ... allow the legs to rest at night, with a completely relaxed and gentle feeling ... ... Imagine that everything important is done during the day, everything important on the outside and, above all, everything important inside, in your feelings ... ... and the legs are allowed to rest in peace at night ... ... Imagine that your conscious mind recognizes your signals and all your deep feelings much better and handles everything important during the day together with you ... ... Imagine that everything important is already done during the day and at night you no longer have to fight and not run, not hurry, and the legs are allowed to rest ... ... Just imagine it with your new path ... ... with a path only you know, subconscious of ... [Client's first name] ... Test whether this path succeeds without leg restlessness ... ...

Test whether your new path with calm legs at night succeeds and show me a signal ... ...

+++ End of Variant 1 +++

+++ Variant 2: Full Body Restlessness, Movement Restlessness at Night +++

... ... Subconscious and conscious mind together ... ... and imagine that you ... ... subconscious of... [Client's first name] ... allow your body to rest at night, with a completely calm feeling ... ... Imagine that everything important is done during the day, everything important on the outside and, above all, everything important inside, in your feelings ... ... and your body is allowed to rest at night, is allowed to recover for the next day ... ... Imagine that your conscious mind recognizes your signals and all your deep feelings much better and handles everything important during the day together with you ... ... Imagine that everything important is already done during the day and at night you no longer have to fight and not exert any effort ... ... your body is finally allowed to rest ... ... Just imagine it with your new path ... ... with a path only you know, subconscious of ...

[Client's first name] … Test whether this path succeeds with complete calmness of the body … … Test whether your new path succeeds and show me a signal … …

+++ End of Variant 2 +++

… if yes … Excellent, your new path succeeds, and it succeeds without restlessness at night … … … if no … It is not yet the best path … … Find another good path of renewal and peace and show me with the yes finger as soon as you have found another path without restlessness … … [Wait for yes finger or repeat until shown! Don't worry, this happens after at most three tries!] … … Excellent, your new path succeeds without restlessness at night … …

… Subconscious of … [Client's first name] … You see that we are making an effort together to understand you and to help you … … The conscious mind and I … … And we will continue to do so, and I promise you that the conscious mind will continue to make an effort to understand your signals and messages … … That's what the conscious mind does for you … … What you have to do is use your new path without restlessness. Only if there is absolutely no other way, do you briefly use the restlessness, just very briefly … … Agreed? … … [A no does not come here anymore] … … Then now set everything up inside you so that from now on, you use this path instead of restlessness … … From now on, everything happens calmly and relaxed at night … … Show me with the yes finger as soon as you're done … … Show me with the yes finger that you have firmly established this new path … … [Wait for yes finger] … …

… … Good, it has succeeded … … You, subconscious of … [Client's first name] … can thoroughly test your new time without nighttime restlessness until we see each other again … … and if your new path works so well, you can keep it forever or even expand and optimize it … … Then you can make the body even calmer and make sleep at night even deeper and more pleasant … …

Distribution, publication, and copying in any form are prohibited and subject to damages.

All Titles in the Series

Volume 1: Smoking Cessation
Volume 2: Anxiety and Restlessness
Volume 3: Burnout
Volume 4: Reducing Overweight
Volume 5: Coping with the Past
Volume 6: Suicidal Thoughts and Attempts
Volume 7: Psycho-Oncology
Volume 8: Obsessions and Tics
Volume 9: Self-Confidence and Decision-Making
Volume 10: Grief Work
Volume 11: Psychosomatics
Volume 12: Chronic Pain
Volume 13: Depressive Thoughts
Volume 14: Panic Attacks
Volume 15: Domestic Violence, Victim Support
Volume 16: Post-Traumatic Stress
Volume 17: Exam Anxiety and Stage Fright
Volume 18: Anti-Violence Training, Offender Support
Volume 19: Addiction Tendencies
Volume 20: Social Phobia and Fear of Contact
Volume 21: Nail Biting
Volume 22: Self-Awareness and Self-Love
Volume 23: Teeth Grinding and Night Clenching
Volume 24: Feelings of Guilt
Volume 25: Fear in Crowds
Volume 26: Fear of Flying, Aviophobia
Volume 27: Fear in Enclosed Spaces, Claustrophobia
Volume 28: Tinnitus, Ear Noises
Volume 29: Fear of Heights
Volume 30: Neurodermatitis

Copying, publishing, and sharing with third parties are only permitted with the written consent of the author. Please observe the notes on copyright and usage.

Volume 31: Finding Inner Balance
Volume 32: Overcoming Loneliness
Volume 33: Fear of Illness, Hypochondria
Volume 34: Anticipatory Anxiety, Fear of Fear
Volume 35: Jealousy in Relationships
Volume 36: Driving Anxiety
Volume 37: New Start after Separation
Volume 38: Fear of Injections
Volume 39: Heart Anxiety Neurosis
Volume 40: Overcoming Resentment and Anger
Volume 41: Resolving Blockages and Positive Thinking
Volume 42: Stress Reduction, Stress Management
Volume 43: Body Relaxation
Volume 44: Deep Relaxation
Volume 45: Fear of the Dark
Volume 46: Falling Asleep and Staying Asleep
Volume 47: Compulsive Buying
Volume 48: Restless Legs Syndrome
Volume 49: Bulimia
Volume 50: Anorexia
Volume 51: Overcoming Nightmares
Volume 52: Imagined Deformity
Volume 53: Overcoming Distrust, Finding Trust
Volume 54: Processing Failures
Volume 55: Humiliation, Emotional Hurt
Volume 56: Distressing Compassion, Vicarious Suffering
Volume 57: Self-Forgiveness
Volume 58: Self-Awareness, Self-Confidence
Volume 59: Saying No
Volume 60: Assertiveness
Volume 61: Setting Boundaries and Self-Assertion
Volume 62: Decision-Making Ability

Volume 63: Success Orientation
Volume 64: Ruminating, Circular Thinking
Volume 65: Accepting Pregnancy
Volume 66: Birth Preparation
Volume 67: Spiritual Opening
Volume 68: Joy of Life and Inner Lightness
Volume 69: Patience and Inner Peace
Volume 70: Fibromyalgia and Rheumatism
Volume 71: Irritable Bowel Syndrome, Crohn's Disease
Volume 72: Fear of Nausea, Emetophobia
Volume 73: Stuttering and Cluttering, Speech Flow Disorders
Volume 74: Concentration and Knowledge Anchoring
Volume 75: Vitality and Spontaneity
Volume 76: Searching for Meaning and Finding Goals
Volume 77: Life Crises, Life Events
Volume 78: Workaholism, Goal Obsession
Volume 79: Helper Syndrome, Helpless Helpers
Volume 80: Medication Abuse
Volume 81: Gambling Addiction
Volume 82: Internet Addiction, Smartphone Addiction
Volume 83: Hoarding Disorder, Compulsive Collecting
Volume 84: Conspiracy Thoughts, Overvalued Ideas
Volume 85: Fear of Operations and Treatments
Volume 86: Fear of Aging
Volume 87: Travel Anxiety
Volume 88: Anxiety When Urinating, Paruresis
Volume 89: Fear of Intimacy and Togetherness
Volume 90: Fear of Blushing
Volume 91: Coming Out in Homosexuality
Volume 92: Charisma Training
Volume 93: Migraines and Chronic Headaches
Volume 94: Overcoming Allergies, Bronchial Asthma

Volume 95: Normalizing Blood Pressure
Volume 96: Compulsive Perfectionism
Volume 97: Sports Hypnosis, Motivation
Volume 98: Sports Hypnosis, Performance Enhancement
Volume 99: Determination and Focus
Volume 100: Encountering the Inner Child
Volume 101: Cravings, Binge Eating
Volume 102: Stimulating Metabolism
Volume 103: Bipolar Mood Swings
Volume 104: Borderline, Identity Crises
Volume 105: Hypomania, Euphoria, Mania
Volume 106: Restlessness, Agitation
Volume 107: Nervous Breakdown
Volume 108: Adjustment Disorders
Volume 109: Self-Alienation, Depersonalization
Volume 110: Ending Self-Pity
Volume 111: Primary Gain of Illness
Volume 112: Secondary Gain of Illness
Volume 113: Bullying, Victim Support
Volume 114: Letting Go of Envy and Jealousy
Volume 115: Fear of Spiders, Arachnophobia
Volume 116: Fear of Dogs or Cats
Volume 117: Fear of Strangers, Xenophobia
Volume 118: Excessive Worries, Generalized Anxiety
Volume 119: Strengthening Sense of Responsibility
Volume 120: Unrequited Love, Heartache
Volume 121: Work-Life Balance
Volume 122: Letting Go of Unattainable Goals
Volume 123: Allowing and Accepting Help
Volume 124: Letting Go of Adult Children
Volume 125: Tourette Syndrome
Volume 126: Life Changes and New Starts

Volume 127: Accepting Life in a Wheelchair
Volume 128: Understanding and Overcoming Homesickness
Volume 129: Understanding and Overcoming Wanderlust
Volume 130: Dizziness, Meniere's Disease
Volume 131: Overcoming Aggression
Volume 132: Cutting and Self-Harm
Volume 133: Hair Pulling, Trichotillomania
Volume 134: Postpartum Depression
Volume 135: For Relatives of Dementia Patients
Volume 136: Self-Harm, Artificial Disorders
Volume 137: Activating Self-Healing Powers
Volume 138: Preventing Depression Relapse
Volume 139: Reactive Psychoses, Follow-Up
Volume 140: Obsessive Thoughts and Impulses
Volume 141: Compulsive Checking
Volume 142: Compulsive Counting, Symmetry Obsession
Volume 143: Compulsive Washing, Cleanliness Obsession
Volume 144: Compulsive Questioning
Volume 145: Dissociative Paralysis
Volume 146: Phantom Pain
Volume 147: Overcoming Complaining
Volume 148: Hay Fever, Pollen Allergy
Volume 149: Sexual Abuse, Victim Support
Volume 150: Standing Strong Against Sexism, #metoo
Volume 151: Binge Eating
Volume 152: Overcoming Thoughts of Revenge
Volume 153: Detachment from the Aggressor, Stockholm Syndrome
Volume 154: Courage to Separate
Volume 155: Chronic Fatigue, Exhaustion
Volume 156: Fear of the Future, Existential Anxiety
Volume 157: Excessive Worry About Children
Volume 158: Fear of Failure

Volume 159: Ending Distrust and Control
Volume 160: Dejection, Dysphoria
Volume 161: Boreout, Chronic Boredom
Volume 162: Bipolar Disorders, Relapse Prevention
Volume 163: Mania, Relapse Prevention
Volume 164: Nihilism, Feelings of Worthlessness
Volume 165: Thumb Sucking
Volume 166: Being Brave
Volume 167: Being Proud
Volume 168: Overcoming Shyness
Volume 169: Being Able to Delegate Responsibility
Volume 170: Being Able to Show Emotions
Volume 171: Letting Go of Guilt, Victim Support
Volume 172: Processing Guilt, Offender Support
Volume 173: Mood Swings, Cyclothymia
Volume 174: Lack of Drive, Vital Sadness
Volume 175: Hearing Voices with Reality Reference
Volume 176: Confident Communication
Volume 177: Standing Up for Oneself
Volume 178: Taking New Paths
Volume 179: Confident Job Application
Volume 180: No Longer Being Taken Advantage Of
Volume 181: End of Submissiveness
Volume 182: Depressive Numbness
Volume 183: Mood Drops, Affective Incontinence
Volume 184: Mood Instability
Volume 185: Somatoform Disorders
Volume 186: Stomach Ulcer, Psychosomatic
Volume 187: Accepting Amputation
Volume 188: Overcoming and Letting Go of Hatred
Volume 189: Ending Accusations
Volume 190: Allowing Tears, Being Able to Cry

Volume 191: Finding and Sorting Repressed Feelings
Volume 192: Somatoform Pain
Volume 193: Living Autonomously
Volume 194: Anhedonia, Joylessness
Volume 195: Persistent Sadness
Volume 196: Obesity, Food Addiction
Volume 197: Parents of Abused Children
Volume 198: Letting Go and Letting Be
Volume 199: Childhood Sexual Abuse
Volume 200: Fear of Loss

www.ingramcontent.com/pod-product-compliance
Lightning Source LLC
Chambersburg PA
CBHW030449220526
45464CB00006B/2458